This book was compiled by Daniel Melehi
with the A.I assistance of Inventabot

<u>Dedication</u>

I hope this helps all of my wonderful
readers achieve all their goals in their
business. And I would like to thank my
wonderful wife for all of her continued
support in all my ventures.

©Daniel Melehi

May 7 2023

Contents

Chapter 1: What Are Anxiety Disorders?

Anxiety is a normal part of life that everyone experiences at some point. It's a feeling of worry, apprehension, or fear about something that may or may not happen in the future. However, when these feelings become persistent, excessive, and interfere with a person's daily life, it may be an indication of an anxiety disorder.

SUBCHAPTER 1.1: SYMPTOMS OF ANXIETY DISORDERS

Anxiety disorders can manifest in different ways, but they all share certain symptoms. Some of the common signs of anxiety disorders include excessive worrying, restlessness, fatigue, trouble sleeping, irritability, difficulty concentrating, sweating, trembling, and increased heart rate. A person may also experience panic attacks, which are episodes of intense fear or discomfort that can lead to physical symptoms like chest pain and shortness of breath.

SUBCHAPTER 1.2: TYPES OF ANXIETY DISORDERS

There are several different types of anxiety disorders, including Generalized Anxiety Disorder (GAD), Panic Disorder, Specific Phobia, Social Anxiety Disorder (SAD), Obsessive-Compulsive Disorder (OCD), and Post-Traumatic Stress Disorder (PTSD). Each type of anxiety disorder has its own set of symptoms and triggers, but they all involve an excessive or unrealistic fear or worry about everyday situations or objects.

SUBCHAPTER 1.3: CAUSES OF ANXIETY DISORDERS

The exact causes of anxiety disorders are not yet understood, but research suggests that a combination of genetic, environmental, and psychological factors may contribute to their development. Trauma, stress, and certain medical conditions can also increase the risk of developing an anxiety disorder. Understanding the root causes of anxiety disorders is important in developing effective treatments.

SUBCHAPTER 1.1: SYMPTOMS OF ANXIETY DISORDERS

Anxiety disorders can manifest in a range of physical, emotional, and cognitive symptoms. Some common symptoms of anxiety disorders include:

1. Excessive worry

One of the most prominent symptoms of anxiety disorders is excessive worry. People with anxiety disorders may worry constantly, and about a wide range of things. They may worry about things that are unlikely to happen, and they may be unable to stop worrying even when they try.

2. Fear and apprehension

People with anxiety disorders may also experience intense fear and apprehension, particularly in certain situations. This fear may be out of proportion to the actual threat posed by the situation.

3. Panic attacks

Another common symptom of anxiety disorders is panic attacks. Panic attacks can involve a range of physical symptoms, including a rapid heartbeat, sweating, trembling, and shortness of breath.

4. Avoidance behavior

People with anxiety disorders may also engage in avoidance behavior, where they avoid certain situations or activities because they fear they will trigger their anxiety.

5. Muscle tension

Anxiety disorders can also cause physical symptoms such as muscle tension. People with anxiety disorders may experience tension headaches, neck and shoulder pain, and other physical discomfort.

6. Sleep disturbances

Sleep disturbances are also common among people with anxiety disorders. They may have trouble falling asleep, staying asleep, or experiencing restful sleep. It's important to note that not everyone with an anxiety disorder will experience all of these symptoms. Additionally, some of these symptoms may be indicative of other mental health conditions, so it's important to seek a proper diagnosis from a qualified mental health professional.

TYPES OF ANXIETY DISORDERS

Anxiety disorders are a group of mental illnesses that are associated with feelings of fear, worry, or apprehension. The following are the most common types of anxiety disorders: 1. Generalized Anxiety Disorder (GAD) - This is a chronic type of anxiety disorder that is characterized by excessive and uncontrollable worry about a variety of different things, such as work, health, family, and finances. 2. Panic Disorder - This type of anxiety disorder involves sudden and unexpected panic attacks, which are characterized by a rapid heartbeat, shortness of breath, dizziness, and intense feelings of fear or dread. 3. Phobias - A phobia is an intense fear of a specific object, situation, or activity. Common phobias include heights, spiders, enclosed spaces, and flying. 4. Social Anxiety Disorder

(SAD) - This type of anxiety disorder is characterized by an intense fear of social situations, such as parties, public speaking, and job interviews. 5. Obsessive-Compulsive Disorder (OCD) - OCD is a type of anxiety disorder that is characterized by recurring, intrusive thoughts (obsessions) and repetitive behaviors (compulsions) that are performed in an attempt to alleviate anxiety. 6. Post-Traumatic Stress Disorder (PTSD) - PTSD is a type of anxiety disorder that can develop after a person experiences a traumatic event, such as military combat, sexual assault, or a natural disaster. Symptoms may include flashbacks, nightmares, and severe anxiety. It is important to remember that anxiety disorders are treatable, and seeking professional help is the first step in managing these conditions.

CHAPTER 1: WHAT ARE ANXIETY DISORDERS?

Subchapter 1.3: Causes of Anxiety Disorders

Anxiety disorders can be caused by a combination of factors. There's no single cause for anxiety disorders, but some factors that may contribute to their development include: **1. Genetics:** Anxiety disorders may be passed down from generation to generation. If you have a family history of anxiety disorders or other mental health disorders, you may be at a higher risk for developing an anxiety disorder yourself. **2. Environmental Factors:** Certain environmental factors and life experiences, such as trauma or chronic stress, may trigger anxiety disorders in some people. **3. Brain Chemistry:** Imbalances in neurotransmitters, which are chemicals in the brain that regulate mood, can contribute to anxiety disorders. Low levels of serotonin in the brain are often associated with anxiety and depression. **4. Medical Conditions:** Certain medical conditions, such as thyroid imbalances or heart disease, can cause symptoms of anxiety. **5. Substance Use and Withdrawal:** Drug and alcohol abuse can trigger anxiety. In addition, withdrawal from drugs or alcohol can cause symptoms of anxiety. It's important to remember that anxiety disorders are not caused by personal weakness, a character flaw, or poor upbringing. Anyone can develop an anxiety disorder, regardless of their background. However, understanding the potential causes of anxiety disorders can help people seek appropriate treatment and reduce their symptoms.

Chapter 2: Understanding Anxiety Disorders

Anxiety disorder is a mental health condition that affects millions of people worldwide. It can be challenging to understand anxiety disorders since the symptoms can vary widely between individuals. However, learning more about anxiety disorders can help you recognize and support those who may be struggling.

SUBCHAPTER 2.1: HOW ANXIETY DISORDERS AFFECT PEOPLE

Living with an anxiety disorder can be challenging. Anxiety can cause physical symptoms, such as increased heart rate, sweating, and difficulty breathing. For others, anxiety can manifest as persistent worry, excessive fear, or intrusive thoughts that interfere with daily activities. Aside from these symptoms, anxiety disorders can also negatively impact emotional and mental well-being. People with anxiety disorders may struggle to maintain relationships, miss out on opportunities, and feel overwhelmed or embarrassed about their experiences.

SUBCHAPTER 2.2: COMMON TRIGGERS FOR ANXIETY ATTACKS

Anxiety attacks, also known as panic attacks, can be triggered by various factors. Some of the most common triggers include stressful events, such as job loss or the end of a relationship. Other triggers may include physical health conditions or a history of trauma or abuse. It is essential to recognize triggers for anxiety attacks, as this can help individuals better manage and prevent episodes from occurring.

SUBCHAPTER 2.3: HOW TO RECOGNIZE ANXIETY DISORDERS IN OTHERS

Recognizing anxiety disorders in other people can be challenging since symptoms can manifest differently between individuals. However, some common warning signs include excessive worry or fear, panic attacks, avoidance of situations or activities, and physical symptoms like sweating or trembling. If you suspect someone you know may be struggling with an anxiety disorder, it is essential to approach them with compassion and support. Encouraging them to seek professional help may be the first step towards recovery. Overall, gaining an understanding of anxiety disorders and how they affect individuals can help us better support those who may be struggling.

HOW ANXIETY DISORDERS AFFECT PEOPLE

Living with anxiety is a daily struggle that can affect every aspect of a person's life. Anxiety disorders are characterized by persistent worry, fear, and physical symptoms that can impair daily activities. Anxiety can be a normal reaction to stress, but when it becomes excessive and disruptive to everyday life, it may be diagnosed as an anxiety disorder. Anxiety disorders can have a profound effect on an individual's emotional, physical, and social health. People with anxiety disorders often struggle with overwhelming feelings of fear and dread, which can lead to physical symptoms such as headaches, muscle tension, and stomach upset. These physical symptoms can affect a person's ability to work, socialize, and engage in everyday activities. In addition to the physical symptoms, anxiety disorders can have a negative impact on a person's emotional well-being. Anxiety can lead to feelings of isolation, shame, and low self-esteem. People with anxiety disorders may feel like they are losing control and may retreat from social situations and relationships to avoid the triggers that cause their anxiety. Anxiety disorders can also create significant challenges in personal and professional relationships. People with anxiety disorders may struggle to communicate their needs effectively, leading to misunderstandings and conflicts. They may also avoid social situations, making it difficult to form new relationships and maintain existing ones. Overall, anxiety disorders are a complex and debilitating condition that can have a significant impact on a person's life. However, with the right treatment and support, people with anxiety disorders can learn to manage their symptoms and live happy, healthy, and fulfilling lives.

SUBCHAPTER 2.2: COMMON TRIGGERS FOR ANXIETY ATTACKS

Anxiety attacks, also known as panic attacks, are sudden and intense surges of fear, panic, and anxiety that can feel overwhelming and debilitating. The onset of an anxiety attack is often unpredictable, and it can occur in seemingly innocuous situations. However, certain triggers can increase the likelihood of experiencing an anxiety attack. Below are some of the most common triggers for anxiety attacks:

1. Stressful life events

Stressful life events such as job loss, a break-up, divorce, financial problems, or moving can trigger anxiety attacks. Major life changes can be unsettling, and uncertainty about the future can trigger feelings of anxiety and panic.

2. Certain medications

Some medications, such as stimulants, decongestants, and some antidepressants, can trigger anxiety attacks. If you experience anxiety after starting a new medication, speak to your doctor about adjusting your dosage or switching to a different medication.

3. Caffeine and alcohol

Caffeine and alcohol can both contribute to feelings of anxiety. Caffeine is a stimulant that can increase heart rate and trigger feelings of nervousness and agitation. Alcohol is a depressant that can worsen anxiety symptoms and trigger a rebound effect once the alcohol wears off.

4. Health conditions

Certain health conditions, such as hypothyroidism, diabetes, and heart disease, can increase the likelihood of experiencing anxiety attacks. If you have a pre-existing health condition and are experiencing anxiety symptoms, speak to your doctor about managing your symptoms.

5. Trauma or PTSD

Traumatic events such as physical or emotional abuse, violence, or an accident can lead to post-traumatic stress disorder (PTSD), which can trigger anxiety attacks. If you have experienced trauma and are experiencing anxiety symptoms, seek support from a therapist or mental health professional who specializes in trauma.

6. Phobias or fears

Specific phobias or fears, such as a fear of spiders or flying, can trigger anxiety attacks. In some cases, exposure to the feared object or situation can elicit intense anxiety symptoms. It's important to remember that everyone's triggers for anxiety attacks are different, and what may cause an anxiety attack in one person may not affect another person. Nevertheless, by understanding some of the most common triggers for anxiety attacks, you can take steps to manage, cope with, and overcome your anxiety symptoms.

HOW TO RECOGNIZE ANXIETY DISORDERS IN OTHERS

Anxiety disorders are not always easy to recognize in others, especially if they are experts at masking their symptoms. However, recognizing the signs of anxiety disorders in others is an essential step in supporting them and encouraging them to seek help. Here are some things to look out for:

Physical Symptoms

One of the most noticeable signs of an anxiety disorder is physical symptoms. These can manifest in various ways, such as an increased heart rate, sweating, fidgeting, and difficulty breathing. Others might complain of stomach aches or headaches. If you notice someone experiencing these symptoms frequently, it might be a sign of an underlying anxiety disorder.

Behavioral Changes

Anxiety disorders can also cause behavioral changes. Someone with anxiety can become withdrawn, avoiding social situations, and engaging in fewer activities. Other behavioral changes can include restlessness, irritability, and difficulty concentrating. These symptoms can impact their work, school, and relationships.

Excessive Worrying

Anxiety disorders can cause individuals to worry excessively. They might worry about day-to-day issues such as paying bills or completing work projects. They can also fixate on more significant life issues, such as their health, finances, or relationships.

Isolation

People with anxiety might prefer to spend time alone, or they might stop attending social events that they previously enjoyed. They might cancel plans or avoid making new ones, preferring the safety and security of being alone.

Conclusion

Recognizing the signs of anxiety disorders in others is the first step towards encouraging them to seek help. If you notice any of the above symptoms in someone you know, it might be time to have an open and supportive conversation about their mental health. Offering them a safe space to discuss their feelings and experience can lead to a positive impact on their mental health.

Coping with Anxiety Disorders

Dealing with anxiety disorders can be overwhelming, but there are several techniques and therapies that can help you manage your symptoms effectively. In this chapter, we will explore some effective coping mechanisms that can help you navigate through challenging times.

SELF-CARE TECHNIQUES FOR MANAGING ANXIETY

One of the most effective ways to manage anxiety is through self-care. Incorporating self-care techniques into your routine can help reduce stress and promote relaxation, ultimately easing anxiety symptoms. Some self-care techniques to consider include:

- Regular exercise

- Meditation
- Yoga or other mindful exercises
- Deep breathing exercises
- Getting enough sleep
- Healthy eating habits and avoiding caffeine or alcohol
- Prioritizing time for activities that bring you joy
- Journaling or expressive writing
- Engaging in hobbies or creative outlets

By taking care of your emotional, physical, and mental health, you are equipping yourself with the tools needed to cope with anxiety.

COGNITIVE BEHAVIORAL THERAPY FOR ANXIETY

Cognitive-behavioral therapy (CBT) is a common therapy technique used to treat anxiety disorders. It focuses on identifying and changing negative thought patterns and behaviors that contribute to anxiety. Through CBT, you will learn how to reframe negative thoughts and beliefs and replace them with positive ones. You will also learn valuable coping skills that can help you manage anxiety symptoms. CBT is typically conducted through weekly sessions and can be done both individually and in a group setting. While CBT can be challenging and intense, it has been found to be highly effective in treating anxiety in the long term.

ALTERNATIVE TREATMENTS FOR MANAGING ANXIETY

There are several alternative therapies that can help manage anxiety, including:

- Acupuncture
- Massage therapy
- Aromatherapy
- Herbal supplements
- Mind-body therapies like hypnotherapy and reflexology

While these therapies are not scientifically proven to cure anxiety disorders, many people find them helpful in managing symptoms. It is always important to consult with your doctor before starting any alternative therapy.

Conclusion

Managing anxiety can be challenging, but there are effective coping mechanisms and therapies that can help ease symptoms. Incorporating self-care techniques into your daily routine, exploring cognitive-behavioral therapy, and trying alternative therapies are all valuable ways to manage anxiety and promote overall health and well-being.

SELF-CARE TECHNIQUES FOR MANAGING ANXIETY

Anxiety can be an overwhelming experience, but there are ways to manage it and get back on track. One of the most important things you can do is take care of yourself. Here are some self-care techniques you can use to manage your anxiety:

1. Practice Relaxation Techniques

One of the best ways to reduce anxiety is to practice relaxation techniques. Techniques such as deep breathing, progressive muscle relaxation, and visualization can help calm your mind and reduce physical symptoms of anxiety. Taking a few minutes to practice these techniques every day can make a big difference.

2. Get Plenty of Sleep

Sleep is essential for maintaining good mental health. Lack of sleep can cause irritability, anxiety, and depression. If you're having trouble sleeping, try creating a relaxing bedtime routine, avoiding caffeine and electronics before bed, and making your bedroom a calm and peaceful environment.

3. Exercise Regularly

Exercise has been shown to be an effective way to manage anxiety. It releases feel-good endorphins, reduces stress hormones, and can help clear your mind and improve your mood. Try to get at least 30 minutes of moderate exercise every day.

4. Eat a Healthy Diet

Eating a healthy, balanced diet can have a big impact on your mental health. Try to eat plenty of fruits, vegetables, whole grains, and lean protein. Avoid processed foods, sugary drinks, and excessive amounts of caffeine and alcohol.

5. Practice Mindfulness

Mindfulness is the practice of paying attention to the present moment without judgment. It can be a helpful tool for managing anxiety and reducing stress. Practicing mindfulness can help you tune out distracting thoughts and focus on the present.

6. Connect with Others

Connection with others is an essential part of mental health. Isolating yourself can make anxiety and depression worse. Seek out supportive friends and family or consider joining a support group. Talking to others who are going through similar experiences can be very helpful.

7. Take Time for Yourself

It's important to make time for things you enjoy. This could be reading a book, taking a walk, or enjoying a hobby. Make sure to schedule time for yourself every day to recharge and focus on self-care. Incorporating these self-care techniques into your daily routine can help you manage your anxiety and improve your overall mental health. Remember, managing anxiety is a journey, and it's important to be patient and kind to yourself along the way.

SUBCHAPTER 3.2: COGNITIVE BEHAVIORAL THERAPY FOR ANXIETY

Cognitive Behavioral Therapy (CBT) is a widely used therapy for the treatment of anxiety disorders. It is a type of psychotherapy that focuses on changing negative thought patterns and behaviors that contribute to anxiety. The goal of CBT is to help individuals learn new skills and coping mechanisms to effectively manage their anxiety. CBT has been shown to be effective in treating various anxiety disorders, including generalized anxiety disorder, panic disorder, obsessive-compulsive disorder, and social anxiety disorder. It typically involves weekly sessions with a therapist and the use of tools such as cognitive restructuring and exposure therapy. Cognitive restructuring involves identifying negative and irrational thoughts that contribute to anxiety and replacing them with more positive and realistic ones.

This involves challenging negative beliefs and learning to think more objectively. Exposure therapy involves gradually exposing the individual to feared objects or situations in a controlled environment, to reduce fear and anxiety over time. CBT for anxiety typically lasts for 12-20 weeks, depending on the severity of the anxiety and the individual's response to treatment. It is important to note that CBT may not work for everyone, and it may take time to see improvements. However, with consistent practice and effort, CBT can be an effective tool for managing anxiety. If you are interested in CBT for anxiety, it is important to find a licensed therapist who specializes in this type of therapy. They can work with you to develop a personalized treatment plan and help you to overcome your anxiety. Remember, it's never too late to seek help and start down the path to recovery.

ALTERNATIVE TREATMENTS FOR MANAGING ANXIETY

While traditional therapy, medication, and self-care techniques are effective methods for managing anxiety, alternative treatments can also be useful. Here are some types of alternative treatments you may want to consider:

1. Yoga

Practicing yoga can help reduce anxiety symptoms. This ancient practice combines physical postures, breathing techniques, and meditation to calm the mind and body. Many people find yoga to be a helpful way to manage their anxiety.

2. Acupuncture

Acupuncture has been used in Traditional Chinese Medicine for centuries to treat various health conditions, including anxiety. Acupuncture involves the insertion of tiny needles into specific points on the body to promote healing and balance. While the mechanism behind acupuncture's effectiveness is not entirely understood, many people report feeling more relaxed after undergoing acupuncture treatment.

3. Massage Therapy

Massage therapy can be an excellent way to relax and relieve anxiety. Therapeutic massage involves the application of pressure to specific areas of the body, providing a soothing and calming effect. Many people find massage therapy to be a helpful adjunct to other anxiety management techniques.

4. Herbal Remedies

Herbs such as chamomile, lavender, and valerian root have natural calming properties that can help reduce anxiety symptoms. These herbs can be taken in various forms, including teas, supplements, or aromatherapy oils.

5. Mindfulness Meditation

Mindfulness meditation involves paying attention to the present moment without judgment. This practice can be an effective way to manage anxiety by developing the ability to focus on the present moment rather than worry about the past or future. While alternative treatments can be useful for managing anxiety, it's important to discuss them with a healthcare professional to ensure they are safe and appropriate for your individual needs. Additionally, it's essential to remember that alternative treatments should not be used as a replacement for traditional therapy or medication but rather as a complement to other anxiety management techniques. Don't hesitate to explore and experiment with different methods until you find what works best for you.

Chapter 4: Overcoming Anxiety Disorders

Anxiety disorders can make people feel overwhelmed and hopeless. However, it is important to remember that anxiety disorders are treatable. In this chapter, we will discuss strategies and tools for overcoming anxiety disorders.

SUBCHAPTER 4.1: HOW TO DEAL WITH ANXIETY ATTACKS

Anxiety attacks can be terrifying and overwhelming. However, there are some ways to deal with them. One effective way is to practice deep breathing. Inhale slowly through your nose and exhale slowly through your mouth. This can help slow down your breathing and decrease your heart rate. Another technique is called grounding. Focus on your senses and describe what you see, hear, feel, and smell around you. This can help pull you out of the anxious thoughts that are causing the attack. It is also important to avoid alcohol and caffeine, which can worsen anxiety symptoms. Instead, try drinking chamomile tea, which has natural calming properties.

SUBCHAPTER 4.2: HOW TO BUILD RESILIENCE AND OVERCOME ANXIETY

Resilience is the ability to bounce back from difficult situations and challenges. Building resilience can help people overcome anxiety disorders. One way to build resilience is to engage in regular exercise and physical activity. Exercise releases endorphins, which are natural mood-boosters. Another way to build resilience is to practice gratitude. Make a list of three things you are thankful for each day. This can help shift your focus to positive things in your life, rather than negative. It is also important to practice self-compassion. Treat yourself with kindness and understanding, rather than harsh judgment. You deserve to be treated with kindness and respect, especially from yourself.

SUBCHAPTER 4.3: LIVING WITH ANXIETY DISORDERS: TIPS FOR A HAPPY, HEALTHY LIFE

Living with an anxiety disorder can be challenging, but there are ways to live a happy and healthy life. One tip is to practice mindfulness. Mindfulness involves paying attention to the present moment with acceptance and non-judgment. This can help reduce anxiety and increase overall well-being. Another tip is to maintain a healthy lifestyle. Eat a balanced diet, get enough sleep, and avoid drugs and alcohol. These healthy habits can support overall mental health and well-being. It is also important to cultivate a support network. Surround yourself with people who support and encourage you. Join a support group, talk to a therapist, or confide in a trusted friend or family member. Remember, overcoming anxiety disorders takes time and effort. Be patient and kind to yourself, and celebrate small victories along the way. With the right tools and support, it is possible to live a happy and fulfilling life with an anxiety disorder.

HOW TO DEAL WITH ANXIETY ATTACKS

When you suffer from an anxiety disorder, you may experience anxiety attacks or panic attacks. An anxiety attack is an intense feeling of fear or distress that often comes unexpectedly. These attacks can be overwhelming and can impact your daily life. Here are some tips on how to deal with anxiety attacks effectively:

Recognize the signs of an anxiety attack

It's important to recognize the physical and emotional symptoms of an anxiety attack. Common signs include rapid heartbeat, excessive sweating, shortness of breath, trembling or shaking, feeling lightheaded or faint, and a sense of impending doom. Once you recognize these symptoms as an anxiety attack, you can start to take steps to manage it.

Practice deep breathing

Deep breathing is an effective technique to help calm your body and mind during an anxiety attack. Take slow, deep breaths in through your nose and out through your mouth. Count to five as you inhale, hold your breath for five seconds, then slowly exhale for five seconds. Repeat this for several minutes until your body begins to relax.

Use grounding techniques

Grounding techniques can help you stay present and focused during an anxiety attack. You can try counting backwards from 100, focusing on objects in your environment, or simply repeating a calming phrase to yourself, such as "I am safe and in control".

Challenge your thoughts

Anxiety attacks are often triggered by negative or irrational thoughts. Challenge these thoughts by asking yourself if they are realistic or helpful. Try to reframe the way you are thinking by focusing on positive outcomes or realistic solutions.

Seek professional help

If you are experiencing frequent or severe anxiety attacks, it's essential to seek professional help. A therapist can help you identify triggers and develop coping strategies. In addition, medication may be prescribed by a doctor to help manage your anxiety. By using these techniques, you can learn to manage and overcome anxiety attacks. Remember that it's normal to feel anxious at times, but with the right tools and support, you can live a happy, healthy life.

HOW TO BUILD RESILIENCE AND OVERCOME ANXIETY

Anxiety disorders can be debilitating, affecting every aspect of a person's life. However, it is not a life sentence, and there are steps you can take to build resilience and overcome anxiety. Here are some tips to help you feel more in control and reduce the symptoms of anxiety:

Practice Relaxation Techniques

Relaxation techniques like deep breathing, progressive muscle relaxation, and visualization can reduce anxiety symptoms and help you feel more relaxed. Practicing these techniques when you feel anxious can help you feel more in control of your body and your thoughts.

Exercise Regularly

Regular exercise has many mental health benefits, including reducing anxiety symptoms. Exercise releases endorphins, which are natural mood boosters. Exercise can also help you sleep better, which can reduce anxiety symptoms.

Eat a Balanced Diet

Maintaining a healthy diet can support your mental health. Eating a balanced diet with plenty of fruits, vegetables, whole grains, and lean proteins can help provide your body with the essential nutrients it needs to function properly.

Create a Support Network

Talking to trusted friends, family, or a support group can help you feel less alone and provide emotional support. Creating a support network can also help you better manage stress and anxiety.

Practice Mindfulness

Mindfulness involves paying attention to the present moment and accepting it without judgment. Practicing mindfulness can help reduce anxiety by interrupting anxious thoughts and promoting relaxation. Mindfulness techniques can involve breathing exercises, body scans, and meditation.

Get Professional Help

If your anxiety symptoms are severe or interfering with your daily life, seeking help from a mental health professional is essential. A therapist can help you identify triggers and develop coping skills to reduce anxiety symptoms. In some cases, medication may also be recommended to help manage anxiety. Building resilience and overcoming anxiety is possible, but it takes time and effort. By practicing relaxation techniques, exercise, eating a balanced diet, creating a support network, practicing mindfulness, and seeking professional help when needed, you can manage your anxiety symptoms and live a happy, healthy life.

LIVING WITH ANXIETY DISORDERS: TIPS FOR A HAPPY, HEALTHY LIFE

Living with anxiety disorders can be a challenging experience, but with the right strategies in place, you can still lead a happy and healthy life. Here are some tips for managing and coping with anxiety disorders:

1. Practice self-care:

Self-care is crucial for everyone, but it's especially important for those living with anxiety disorders. Practicing good self-care techniques can help you reduce stress, improve your mood, and maintain your physical wellbeing. Some self-care techniques for managing anxiety can include practicing meditation or deep breathing exercises, getting regular exercise, getting enough sleep, eating a healthy diet, and taking breaks from stressful situations when needed.

2. Create a support system:

Having a good support system in place can help you feel more connected and less isolated. Consider joining a support group for individuals with anxiety disorders, speaking with a trusted friend or family member, or seeking the help of a mental health professional. Remember that it's okay to ask for help and that seeking support does not make you weak.

3. Develop coping mechanisms:

Coping mechanisms can help you manage anxiety symptoms when they arise. Examples of coping mechanisms can include journaling, practicing mindfulness, engaging in creative activities, or finding relaxation techniques that work for you. You may need to experiment with different coping mechanisms to find what works best for you.

4. Set realistic goals:

Anxiety disorders can make it difficult to achieve goals or make progress towards them. It's important to set realistic goals for yourself and to break larger goals down into smaller, more manageable steps. Celebrate your successes along the way, no matter how small they may seem.

5. Limit stressors:

While it's impossible to eliminate all stressors from your life, it's important to look for ways to limit them. This could mean setting boundaries with work or personal commitments, learning how to say "no" when you need to, or finding ways to delegate tasks to others. By implementing these strategies, you can learn to manage your anxiety symptoms and lead a happier, healthier life. Remember to be patient with yourself and to seek help when you need it.

Chapter 5: Seeking Help for Anxiety Disorders

Anxiety is a normal human emotion, but it becomes a problem when it interferes with daily life. For people who have anxiety disorders, seeking professional help can make a huge difference in managing symptoms and improving their quality of life. If you think you have an anxiety disorder and need help, this chapter can guide you on where to start seeking professional help.

SUBCHAPTER 5.1: HOW TO FIND A GOOD THERAPIST

One important step in seeking help for anxiety disorders is to find the right therapist. Here are some things to consider when looking for a therapist:

Evidence-Based Treatment Approaches:

Find a therapist practicing evidence-based treatments for anxiety disorders. These treatment approaches are backed by scientific research and have been proven to be effective. Some common evidence-based treatments are Cognitive-Behavioral Therapy (CBT), Acceptance and Commitment Therapy (ACT), Exposure Therapy, and Mindfulness-Based Stress Reduction (MBSR).

Qualifications and Specialization:

Make sure your therapist has the appropriate qualifications and experience to treat anxiety disorders. Look for a licensed mental health professional with a specialization in anxiety disorders. This includes Psychologists, Psychiatrists, and Clinical Social Workers.

Compatibility:

It is equally important to feel comfortable with your therapist. Don't be afraid to shop around until you find the right one. Finding a good therapist can be a bit like dating. It can take some time, and it may take a few sessions to get a feel for a therapist's style and whether you click.

SUBCHAPTER 5.2: MEDICATIONS FOR ANXIETY: WHAT YOU NEED TO KNOW

Medication can be an effective treatment for anxiety disorders if prescribed and managed correctly. Here are some things to know about medications for anxiety:

Types of Medications:

There are different types of medications prescribed for anxiety disorders. The main ones include Antidepressants, Benzodiazepines, Beta Blockers, and

Anticonvulsants. Antidepressants are the most commonly prescribed medication for anxiety disorders.

Adverse Effects:

All medications can have side effects, so it's important to talk with your doctor about any concerns you might have. Some people may experience symptoms such as dizziness, nausea, weight gain or loss, or sexual dysfunction.

Consultation:

If you're interested in taking medication for your anxiety disorder, it's important to talk with a qualified healthcare professional who can evaluate your symptoms, diagnose your condition, and prescribe the appropriate medication.

SUBCHAPTER 5.3: SUPPORT GROUPS FOR ANXIETY: FINDING HELP AND HOPE

In addition to receiving professional help, support groups can be an excellent way to get the support and encouragement necessary to manage anxiety disorders. Here's how to find a good support group:

Online:

There are many online support groups available for people struggling with anxiety disorders. These groups can be accessed from the comfort of your home at any time. You can find these online support groups on websites or social media platforms.

In-person:

You can also find local in-person support groups in your community. You can start by reaching out to local clinics, community centers, and mental health organizations.

Psychological Help:

It's important to remember that support groups are not a substitute for professional help. They can serve as an addition to your treatment but are not a replacement. A mental health professional understands anxiety disorders deeply and will properly diagnose and treat it, so it's important to seek professional help if you feel overwhelmed.

Conclusion:

Seeking help for anxiety disorders is necessary for individuals to live a quality life, so it's important to know where to start. Finding a good therapist, considering medications, and support groups are all great options to consider. By taking action, seeking professional help, and finding supportive communities, you can reclaim your life from anxiety.

HOW TO FIND A GOOD THERAPIST

Finding a good therapist can be a challenging task, but it's an essential step towards managing and treating anxiety disorders. Here are a few things you can keep in mind while searching for a therapist.

Consider Your Preferences

The first thing to do is to consider your preferences. Consider the type of therapist you want to work with, such as a cognitive-behavioral therapist or a psychoanalyst. Also, think about whether you want to work with a male or female therapist, or whether you want to make use of telemental health services.

Ask for Referrals

One of the best ways to find a good therapist is by asking for referrals from friends and family. If you know someone who has worked with a therapist before and had a positive experience, they might be able to recommend someone to you.

Check Credentials

Another important factor to consider is the therapist's credentials. Look for a therapist who has a license to practice in your state and who has undergone the necessary training and education required to treat anxiety disorders. You can check the therapist's credentials on the website of your state's regulatory board.

Interview the Therapist

Once you've found a few therapists who seem like a good fit, reach out to them and schedule an initial consultation. This consultation will give you an opportunity to ask questions and get to know the therapist before committing to treatment. Some questions you might consider asking include: - What is your experience treating anxiety disorders? - What is your therapeutic approach? - How long do you typically work with patients? - What is your fee structure? - Do you accept insurance?

Trust Your Gut

Finally, as you search for a therapist, remember to trust your gut. If you have a negative gut feeling about a particular therapist, it's probably best to move on and find someone who feels like a better fit. Building trust and establishing a good relationship with your therapist is crucial to the success of your treatment. Overall, finding a good therapist may take some effort and time, but it's a crucial investment towards managing your anxiety disorder. Remember to consider your preferences, ask for referrals, check credentials, interview the therapist, and trust your gut.

SUBCHAPTER 5.2:
MEDICATIONS FOR ANXIETY: WHAT YOU NEED TO KNOW

Anxiety disorders can often be treated with medication, in combination with therapy and lifestyle changes. It's important to note that each person's experience with medication is different, and what works for one person may not work for another. It's always important to work closely with a healthcare provider to determine the best course of treatment for you. There are several different classes of medications that can be used to treat anxiety disorders. One of the most commonly prescribed classes of medications are selective serotonin reuptake inhibitors (SSRIs). These medications work by increasing levels of the neurotransmitter serotonin in the brain, which can improve mood and reduce symptoms of anxiety. Another class of medications that may be used to treat anxiety disorders are benzodiazepines. These medications work by enhancing the activity of a neurotransmitter called gamma-aminobutyric acid (GABA), which can help to reduce feelings of anxiety and promote relaxation. However, benzodiazepines can be habit-forming and may have side effects such as dizziness, drowsiness, and impaired coordination. Other medications, such as beta blockers and antipsychotics, may also be used to treat anxiety disorders in some cases. Beta blockers can help to reduce physical symptoms of anxiety, such as heart palpitations and tremors, while antipsychotics may be used in more severe cases of anxiety disorder or when other treatments have not been effective. As with any medication, there are potential side effects to consider when taking medications for anxiety disorder. It's important to discuss these risks with your healthcare provider and closely monitor any changes in symptoms or side effects while taking these medications. It's also important to remember that medication may not be the best option for everyone and should always be used as part of a comprehensive treatment plan that includes therapy and lifestyle changes. Overall, medications can be an effective tool in treating anxiety disorders, but they should always be used in conjunction with other treatments and under the guidance of a healthcare provider.

SUPPORT GROUPS FOR ANXIETY: FINDING HELP AND HOPE

Living with anxiety disorders can be overwhelming and isolating, but finding a supportive community can make a big difference in managing symptoms and improving overall well-being. One such community is support groups, which provide a safe space to share experiences, learn coping strategies, and connect with others who understand what you're going through.

What are Anxiety Support Groups?

Anxiety support groups are usually led by a mental health professional or a trained volunteer who has personal experience with anxiety disorders. The groups can take place in-person or online and typically consist of small groups of individuals who come together to discuss and share their experiences.

How Can Support Groups Help?

Joining an anxiety support group can help you in several ways:

- Understand that you're not alone - knowing that others are also experiencing anxiety can help you feel less isolated and alone.
- Learn from others - sharing experiences and hearing how others have been able to cope can provide you with new strategies for managing your own anxiety.
- Receive support and validation - support groups provide a safe and

non-judgmental space to talk about your anxiety and receive validation and support from others who get it.

- Gain a sense of empowerment - hearing how others have overcome their anxiety and regained control of their lives can inspire you to take steps to do the same.
- Improve overall well-being - being part of a supportive community can improve overall mental and emotional well-being.

How to Find a Support Group for Anxiety?

Finding the right support group for you may take some time and effort. Here are some tips to get started:

- Talk to your therapist or mental health provider - they may know of local support groups or online communities that may be helpful.
- Search online - there are several online support groups for anxiety disorders, and many are free and open to anyone.

- Check with non-profit organizations - non-profit organizations such as NAMI (National Alliance on Mental Illness) may offer support groups for anxiety disorders.
- Ask in online forums - online forums, such as Reddit, may be a good place to ask for recommendations or connect with others who may know of helpful resources.

Conclusion

Support groups provide a valuable resource for individuals living with anxiety disorders. They offer a safe and supportive space to share experiences and learn new coping strategies. If you're struggling with anxiety, don't hesitate to reach out and join a support group. Remember, there is hope, and there is help available!

Breaking the Stigma Around Anxiety Disorders

Anxiety disorders are often misunderstood and stigmatized by society, which can make it difficult for those who suffer from them to seek help or feel accepted. In this chapter, we will explore the common misconceptions surrounding anxiety disorders and discuss the ways in which we can work to break down the stigma and promote open communication about mental health.

ADDRESSING STIGMA AND MISCONCEPTIONS ABOUT ANXIETY

One of the biggest barriers to seeking help for anxiety disorders is the social stigma attached to mental illness. Many people still believe that anxiety disorders are a sign of weakness or that individuals who suffer from them should simply "get over it." These misconceptions can be harmful and hinder those who need help from seeking it. It is important to address and challenge these misconceptions. Anxiety disorders are not the result of a person being weak or lazy. They are a real and serious mental health condition that requires treatment, just like any other illness. It's essential that we educate ourselves and others on the facts surrounding anxiety disorders to break down the stigma.

ENCOURAGING OPEN COMMUNICATION ABOUT MENTAL HEALTH

Breaking the stigma surrounding anxiety disorders starts with open communication. When we talk openly about mental health, we break down the societal barriers that make it difficult for individuals to seek help. If we can create a culture where speaking about anxiety and other mental health issues is normalized, we can help individuals feel more comfortable seeking treatment and support. We can start by sharing our own stories and experiences with anxiety and encouraging others to do the same. We can also work towards creating safe spaces where individuals can feel comfortable talking about mental health without fear of judgement or discrimination.

HELPING OTHERS WITH ANXIETY DISORDERS: HOW TO BE A SUPPORTIVE FRIEND OR FAMILY MEMBER

Support from friends and family can be essential for someone suffering from an anxiety disorder. Here are some ways you can support your loved one:

Be a Good Listener

Many individuals with anxiety disorders may just need someone to listen to them. Try to let your loved one vent without interrupting or trying to solve their problem.

Show Empathy

It's important to validate your loved one's feelings and show empathy towards them. Let them know that you're there for them and that you understand what they're going through.

Encourage Them to Get Help

If your loved one is struggling with an anxiety disorder, encourage them to seek professional help. This can involve helping them find a therapist or offering to accompany them to appointments. In conclusion, breaking the stigma surrounding anxiety disorders is essential to promoting open communication and encouraging individuals to seek help. By addressing and challenging misconceptions, encouraging open communication, and being supportive of loved ones, we can work towards creating a society that is more accepting and understanding of mental health struggles.

ADDRESSING STIGMA AND MISCONCEPTIONS ABOUT ANXIETY

It's a sad reality that many people still associate mental health issues with weakness, and anxiety disorders are no exception. This can make it very difficult for people who suffer from anxiety disorders to speak out about their condition and seek the help they need. In this subchapter, we will explore the impact of stigma and misconceptions surrounding anxiety disorders and how we can work together to break down the barriers to seeking help. One of the biggest misconceptions surrounding anxiety disorders is that they are just a minor issue, or that people who suffer from anxiety just need to "snap out of it" or "get over it." However, anxiety disorders are a real and serious health issue that can have a major impact on a person's quality of life. Anxiety can lead to physical symptoms, such as headaches and muscle tension, as well as psychological symptoms, such as constant worry and fear. Stigma can also be a major barrier to seeking help for anxiety. Unfortunately, many people still associate mental health issues with weakness or a lack of willpower, which can make it very difficult for people who suffer from anxiety to speak out and seek treatment. This can be especially true in certain cultures or communities, where mental health issues may be seen as taboo or shameful. So, how can we break down these barriers and address the stigma and misconceptions surrounding anxiety disorders? Education is key. The more we can learn about anxiety disorders and how they impact people's lives, the more we can help break down the myths and stereotypes that can prevent people from seeking help. We need to encourage open discussions about mental health, and create safe and supportive environments where people feel comfortable opening up about their struggles. Another important step is to seek out credible and accurate information about anxiety disorders. There is so much misinformation out there about mental health issues, and it can be overwhelming to try to separate fact from fiction. One great resource for learning more about anxiety disorders is the National Institute of Mental Health (NIMH), which offers a wealth of information and resources for people who are looking to learn more about anxiety disorders and how to seek treatment. Finally, we need to continue to advocate for increased access to mental health resources and support. Unfortunately, many people still face significant barriers to accessing mental health treatment, whether due to cost, availability, or other factors. We need to work together to create a more equitable and accessible mental healthcare system, so that everyone who needs help can receive the care and support they deserve. In conclusion, addressing the stigma and misconceptions surrounding anxiety disorders is an essential step in promoting mental health and wellness. By educating ourselves and others, seeking out accurate and reliable information, and advocating for increased access to mental health resources and support, we can work together to break down the barriers to seeking help and create a brighter, more compassionate future for everyone affected by anxiety disorders.

ENCOURAGING OPEN COMMUNICATION ABOUT MENTAL HEALTH

One of the biggest obstacles for those dealing with mental health issues is the stigma around it. Many people fear judgement or rejection if they speak up about their struggles. However, it is vital that we encourage open communication about mental health to break down this stigma and provide much-needed support. One way to start is by showing empathy and understanding towards those who do open up to us. It's crucial to avoid judgement and instead offer support and validation. One can start by responding with phrases such as

"I am here for you" or "Thank you for trusting me with this information." Talking openly about one's own mental health struggles can also help normalize the conversation. It can create a safe space for others to feel comfortable sharing their own experiences as well. However, this can be challenging for some people, and it's important to only share as much as one feels comfortable with. In addition to personal conversations, it can also be helpful to encourage open communication on a larger scale. This can involve advocating for mental health resources in schools and workplaces or supporting mental health campaigns online. By promoting education and awareness about mental health, we can help break down the barriers to communication and provide a support system for those in need. Overall, encouraging open communication about mental health is crucial for breaking the stigma and providing support to those in need. By showing empathy, sharing personal experiences, and advocating for mental health resources, we can create a more compassionate and understanding society.

9 798394 642012